- # **Sample Exercise #1**

<u>Wall pushups</u>

This is a modified version of the regular push up. It is less challenging than the regular version but it can still strengthen your arms, chest and shoulders. Find a flat wall near you and stand at an arm's length from it.

Face the wall and lean forward. Place your palms against the wall at shoulder height. Bend your elbow as you lean in. Count to four as you move your body towards the wall. Pause for few seconds then push your body back up. Work up to a total of 10 repetitions and 2 sets. Make sure that you do not arch your back.

- # **Sample Exercise #2**

<u>Cycling/Biking</u>

Riding a bike can be a good exercise for seniors. It can also double as an effective means of transportation. Some seniors may find a recumbent bike more comfortable. You can also adjust the seat and add padding if necessary. Seniors who experience balancing problems may opt for a three wheeled bike instead. Indoor stationary bikes, upright and recumbent, are available commercially if you don't want to ride outside.

But, if you wish to ride your bike outdoors, be very cautious in choosing your route most especially if you have sight impairment. You should also consider cycling in a nearby park instead of on roads with traffic.

- # **Sample Exercise #3**

Flexibility Exercise

Shoulder and upper arm rise

Stand with your feet apart. Hold one end of a towel with your one hand. Bend your arm to drape the towel on your back. Reach behind you and grasp the other end with your other arm. Stretch your shoulder by pulling the towel down with your one arm. Reverse the movement and repeat 5 times.

Upper body stretch

Stand facing the wall. You should be an arm's length away from the wall. Lean your body forward and place your hand flat against the wall on chest level. Make sure that your back is straight. Slowly walk your hands up the wall until it is above your head. Repeat 5 times.

• Sample Question Answered

What is weight loss plateau and how do I overcome it?

Weight loss plateau occurs when your body stops losing weight even if you are still continuing your fitness program. You will eventually hit a plateau once your body starts to adapt to your fitness routine. You can start increasing the intensity and duration of your exercise and altering your diet to start losing weight again.

Over Age 60 Senior Body Manual
Muscle and Flexibility Secrets in 4 Stages

By
Jack Sampson

ISBN-13: 978-1502596703

ISBN-10: 1502596709

Introduction

I want to thank you and congratulate you for purchasing this book, "Over Age 60 Senior Body Manual".

This book contains proven steps and strategies on how to exercise if you are over 60.

A person's physical and mental capabilities can decline because of age. However, people over 60 can still manage to look and feel young by incorporating healthy habits into their daily routine.

As you get older, it becomes more important to maintain an exercise habit. Different types of exercise can strengthen your body and make it more resistant to disease and external injuries. Studies also show that physical exercise improves cognitive ability for seniors.

Older people may face different challenges when it comes to exercising compared to the general population but are still capable of performing varying levels of exercise. You can start with easy workouts and gradually increase your intensity as your body gets used to it.

It is never too late to start taking care of your body. Exercise and physical activity can help you achieve a healthy body and mind.

Thanks again for downloading this book, I hope you enjoy it!

Disclaimer:

Chapter 1. About Exercise

Regular physical fitness becomes more important as people grow older. Exercise can help boost your energy and maintain your physical independence. Some studies also show that exercise can reverse the signs of aging.

History of Exercise

The history of physical activity can be traced back to the early existence of mankind. Although early humans may not have recognized their activities as 'exercise', still their active lifestyle made them physically stronger and fit. It was around 400 BC when Hippocrates promoted the idea of a healthy diet and exercise as the safest ways to maintain good health. This encouraged people to study in detail the importance and relevance of physical exercise to the human body.

The exact period of the development of various systematic exercise routines to build muscles and burn fat is not clearly known. Some scientists suggest that such physical practices may have originated in Italy, India and Greece during the 9th century where wars and battles were common. The discoveries of stone weights in India and some areas in Europe support these theories.

The more modern exercise routine started to develop during the 18th century when exercises became more streamlined and efficient workout routines started to become popular because of modern medicine and scientific theories. It was also in this period when aerobics, running and weight training evolved. Myths about exercise were debunked by scientific studies and experiments.

In the 19th century, the development in science and technology gave way to the inventions of in-house training equipment like the tread mill, chest and shoulder benches and exercise bikes. Such equipment enabled more people to become physically fit. The number of gyms also increased drastically. The development of the television also inspired the idea of achieving physical fitness. Remember Jack

LaLanne? Many people took their fitness inspiration from celebrities and TV personalities. A few years later, people started using exercise videos for home use.

Benefits of working out

<u>Physical health benefits</u>

Exercise helps older people maintain a healthy weight.

Metabolism naturally slows down because of age and maintaining a healthy weight becomes more challenging. Exercise can help people burn calories to improve overall wellness.

    a) Exercise can reduce the risk of illness.

People over 60 are more susceptible to many diseases because their body is not as strong as it once was. Exercise can prevent many diseases including colon cancer, heart disease, stroke and diabetes.

    b) It enhances mobility and flexibility.

Exercise can help develop a person's flexibility and strength. This can help seniors improve their coordination and balance. Strength training also alleviates chronic conditions like arthritis. Exercise can prevent bone breakage and loss in bone mass. Studies show that strength training can drastically reduce bone loss and help contribute to better balance.

    c) Improved healing

Injuries become harder to heal as people grow older. Regular exercise can speed up the natural healing process by as much as 25%. Exercise can also improve seniors' immunity. A healthy and strong body can fight infection better.

    d) A little goes a long way

When it comes to physical exercise for older people, consistency is much more important than intensity. You do not have to do strenuous physical exercise to reap the benefits. Moderate exercise like walking five days a week can readily produce many benefits.

<u>Mental benefits</u>

    a) Improves quality of life

Studies show that physical activity can produce hormones in the body that reduce stress. Exercise can also result in psychological benefits and help seniors relieve anxiety.

b) Improves your sleep

Poor sleep quality is not a direct result of aging. Sleep is essential for your overall health. Exercise can help people fall asleep faster. It also enables seniors to sleep better.

c) Boosts self-confidence

Engaging in physical exercise can give seniors a sense of independence and can reduce feelings of depression and sadness.

d) Exercise is good for the brain

Exercise is essential to keep your brain active to prevent memory loss and cognitive decline. Exercise can effectively reduce the risk of brain disorders like dementia.

Chapter 2. Improving Fitness by Working Out

Regular exercise provides many benefits for the body. However, there are also drawbacks that you have to be prepared for if you want to make exercise a part of your daily regimen.

Pros and Cons of Working out

Pros

Increase in Energy

An increase in energy levels is one of the best benefits of exercise for elderly people. Exercise can naturally increase your stamina and enable you to perform the needed chores throughout the day. Instead of relying on caffeine for your mid-afternoon boost, try to go for a walk for few minutes and you might be surprised at how energetic you feel afterwards.

Prevent lethargy

The body can respond quickly to physical exercise. Seniors may fear that they don't have enough energy to finish their workout but you will be amazed at how much energy the body actually has. Give it ten minutes and see how your body responds to the exercise. If you still feel tired, you can take a break and rest. More often than not, it gets easier to finish your workout once you have started to increase your blood flow.

Better memory

Senior moments are annoying. Improve your memory by engaging in physical exercise. Just 20 minutes of exercise performed three times a week can improve your cognitive ability.

A positive outlook on life

Seniors who find themselves getting moody can benefit from exercise. Exercise can improve blood flow to the brain and increase serotonin production which reduces stress and eases mood swings. Moderate exercise can also relieve irritability.

Look younger

Increased blood flow and oxygen in the body can improve skin elasticity and prevent wrinkles. Increased oxygenation can also encourage skin cell turnover and helps fight off free radicals and provide you with a youthful glow.

Cons

Increased risk of injury

If you have never engaged in physical exercise before you might not know how to perform various activities properly. This can increase your risk of injury. If you are unsure, try to contact a personal trainer who can correct your posture and design a specific program for you.

Indulging in the halo effect

Exercise can suppress your appetite but some people may use this as an excuse to indulge in unhealthy food. Once you start an exercise program, be careful that you do not derail all your efforts by eating more. Keep in mind that you should exercise to improve your health and as a benefit, lose some weight.

Change relationships

This is something that people rarely think about. However, if you try a new healthy lifestyle other people in your life may not support you immediately. Dedicating some of your time engaging in physical fitness can affect some of your relationships. To some people, your dedication to daily exercise can appear vain or even selfish. Your friends might think that you prefer to go to the gym instead of having some fun with them. Be sure to invite other people to participate in your workout if you can. Physical activities like running, aerobic classes and sports can also be a social experience which you can enjoy with your family and friends. Use this as an opportunity to create a healthy lifestyle and strengthen your social relationships as well.

Dos and Don'ts for Exercising

Do

Warm up

People tend to neglect warm up as part of their daily exercise routine but you will not be able to reap the full benefits of your exercise if you do not warm up. Try gentle exercise like walking to prepare your body before engaging in rigorous workout.

Stretch more

Stretching is also a part of good exercise routine. It can improve your range of motion and even your flexibility. A good stretching exercise can also reduce the risk of muscles soreness and strain. To get the most of your stretch, do it after your workout while your muscles are still warm.

Bring your own water

If you tend to work out in a gym, bring your own bottle of water and make it a habit to drink regularly even if you are not thirsty. Thirst is usually a signal that you are on your way to dehydration.

Work out just right

Seniors should focus on working out at the just the right amount of intensity to prevent injuries. You should challenge your body enough so that it can change but not too much or you might get hurt.

Don't

Lift too much

While strength training should be included in your routine, you should only start with weights that are appropriate for your fitness level and gradually increase them later on. Lifting to the point where you feel slight discomfort is normal but do not do it to the point of muscle exhaustion.

Eat too much

If you exercise for less than two hours, you would not be needing energy bars and any sport drinks to fuel your workout. Also, some sports bars are very high in calories which can only negate your efforts.

Socialize too much and not exercise enough

Getting social support from common minded peers can give you the motivation you need but don't get carried away. Do not go to the gym to catch up with your friends or you might get distracted about actually working out.

Maintain a plateau

If you do a workout over and over again, your body will start to adapt to it. You might see an initial change at the beginning it you will eventually reap less and less benefits. Incorporating small changes in your workout routine can make your exercise more exciting.

Use spot reduction training

Everyone has their own 'problem spot' which they wish to improve but focusing on a well balanced training program can ensure that you lose weight from all the areas in your body.

Employ improper technique

If you do not know how to use exercise equipment properly, you might confuse caloric burn with mechanical inefficiency. This can lead to injuries. Consider asking gym personnel to do the rounds with you and teach you the basic technique.

Do too much too soon

If you quickly jump into your exercise program, you might hurt yourself. While feeling sore results from an effective work out, working too hard early on can have detrimental effects on motivation especially for older people.

Rules to consider when exercising at a commercial fitness center

1. Clean up after you finish

This is one of the most basic rules at the gym. Make sure to return the weights and equipment to their proper place. Also, always bring a towel to wipe your sweat before it dries on the equipment.

2. Step away from the rack

The rack is almost always located in front of the mirror but this does not mean that you can pick up couple of weights, take few steps back and start lifting the weights. Try to move away from the rack to give way for others to get to the equipment as well.

3. Avoid hoarding the equipment

Do not take up multiple machines or horde a lot of weights. Remember that gym equipment is for everybody to use. If you wish to have free access to all the gym equipment then try to go to the gym during the off hours.

4. Don't do the walking lunges

Most gyms have a walkway that leads to the weight area. Avoid using it as a lane for walking lunges. You can do stationary lunges instead and make sure to get out of the walking path.

5. No reservations

A towel or a water bottle left on equipment does not count as a reservation. Give a chance for other people and use one machine at a time. Do not leave your stuff on a single piece of equipment and walk away to chat with someone.

6. Give people their personal space

Make it a habit to step away from people who are lifting weights. Wait until they have finished their set before engaging them in a conversation.

7. Be alert

Lifting weights and using cardio machines is usually safe but you always have to be aware of your surroundings to ensure safety. Focus on your workout and avoid day dreaming while running on the treadmill.

8. Manage your personal hygiene

Granted, going to the gym is not the same as going to a party so you do not have to spray on a bottle of cologne, but make sure you smell clean when you work out. Shower and use deodorant liberally.

9. Be courteous and friendly

Being nice to others in the gym can go a long way. There is nothing wrong with being courteous and offering a little smile to other people. Apply the Golden Rule.

Chapter 3. Cardio Exercises for People over 60

Regular cardiovascular workout is important for any age group to maintain a healthy heart. Cardiovascular workouts improve oxygen and blood circulation in the body and help ease respiratory problems.

Step by step approach to exercising
1. Choose an activity

The best activities will be the ones that you enjoy doing. Make sure to perform the activities at a moderate intensity level or about 70-80% of your heart rate.

2. Choose the duration of your exercise

Aim for a minimum of 30 minutes of physical exercise each day. You may need to start with just 5 minutes then gradually increase the time once you feel comfortable with the routine.

3. Schedule your workouts

Start by exercising three times a week with rest days in between. You can add more exercise days if you feel that you are ready.

The best methods for a cardio workout

Walking

Walking is a great cardio workout for people over 60 since it requires no special equipment and it allows you to set your own pace. Try to take short walks to increase your heart rate and improve the blood circulation in your legs.

Warm-up

Before going into a vigorous walking program, make sure to warm up the muscles and start slowly. Stand up straight and rotate your arms in a circular motion. This loosens the muscles and gets the blood flowing. You can hold on to a chair or rest your hand on the wall for balance. Practice lifting one foot then the other to prepare your body for the walking exercise.

Set the pace

Before you begin your exercise, understand where you are going. Choose a route that is safe and one that you are familiar with. A course on flat terrain without too many hills is ideal for seniors who are starting a workout program.

Swing your arms back and forth to incorporate arm motion. This can maximize the aerobic benefits of your walk. Set your pace and walk for 5 minutes before you start to increase your speed.

Power walking

A regular walking routine can be the building block to a more advanced cardio exercise. Make sure that you are walking faster than you normally would. You should also be breathing faster but not too labored.

Water exercise

Water exercises can be soothing for people over 60 years old. Water has a therapeutic benefit to the joints and does not place too much stress on them. This makes it beneficial for people with arthritis.

Swimming

Swimming is a classic cardio exercise that can increase your heart rate and can provide an overall work out for your body. It can improve your heart and lung function.

You can enroll in a local swimming gym if you do not know how to swim. Most YMCA fitness centers also have a swimming pool which you can practice on.

Water aerobics

Most people are familiar with aerobic exercises like walking, dancing and step classes. These activities can effectively increase your heart rate and circulation. You can also do these aerobic exercises in the water. Aqua aerobics are conducted on different gyms and fitness centers. You can do various activities like jumping jacks, walking and even dancing. Make sure that you have enough time to warm-up and cool down properly.

Relaxation

Floating in water can be a relaxing exercise for anyone. Submerging your body in a pool of warm water can also ease sore muscles and joints. This activity can also reduce your stress levels while increasing your energy and immunity.

Dance Exercise

Dancing is an effective physical exercise for seniors. Dance therapy can also improve your balance and agility. Dancing encourages seniors to move in different direction. This helps improve their walking speed and stamina.

Zumba

One of the most popular cardio dance exercise is the zumba. There are a lot of fitness centers that offer this class and there are also DVDs if you want to dance in the comfort of your own home. Most zumba exercises for seniors combine slow dance movements and aerobic routines.

Jazz exercise

Jazz exercise combines aerobic exercise and jazz dancing. This is very similar to zumba but it focuses more on strength training and toning the body. Cardio is the main component of this exercise.

Hip hop

Surprisingly, many seniors also enjoy modern dances like hip hop. The upbeat music can be fun and energizing at the same time. It combines a lot of hip movements and aerobic moves.

Belly dancing

Belly dancing can produce the same effects as cardio dance. Belly dancing DVDs are also readily available and there are a lot of centers offering different classes. The main benefit derived from this exercise aside from a cardio workout is that it can effectively tone the core area of the body.

Salsa

Salsa is a great calorie burning exercise which can also be very enjoyable. Salsa is a great dance that requires a partner so you can enjoy it with a friend.

Cycling/Biking exercises

Riding a bike can be a good exercise for seniors. It can also double as an effective means of transportation. Some seniors may find a recumbent bike more comfortable. You can also adjust the seat and add padding if necessary. Seniors who experience balancing problems may opt for a three wheeled bike instead. Indoor stationary bikes, upright and recumbent, are available commercially if you don't want to ride outside.

But, if you wish to ride your bike outdoors, be very cautious in choosing your route most especially if you have sight impairment. You should also consider cycling in a nearby park instead of on roads with heavy traffic.

Chapter 4. Strength Exercises for People over 60

Studies show that strength training can be beneficial for people of all ages. For people over 60 years of age, strength training can effectively relieve chronic conditions like back pain and arthritis.

Stage 1: Easy

Squats

This is a great exercise for strengthening your buttocks, hips and thighs.

Stand with your feet slightly apart. Extend your arms in front of you. Make sure that they are parallel to the ground. You can lean forward a little bit. Lower your body in a slow and controlled motion until you reach a near sitting position.

Pause and slowly rise back up. Remember to keep your back straight and your knees over your ankles. Repeat this for 10 times. You can rest for a minute before repeating another set. Make sure that you do not lean too far or place your toes too far forward.

Wall pushups

This is a modified version of the regular push up. It is less challenging than the regular version but it can still strengthen your arms, chest and shoulders. Find a flat wall near you and stand at an arm's length from it.

Face the wall and lean forward. Place your palms against the wall at shoulder height. Bend your elbow as you lean in. Count to four as you move your body towards the wall. Pause for few seconds then push your body back up. Work up to a total of 10 repetitions and 2 sets. Make sure that you do not arch your back.

Toe stands

If you find it difficult to walk, try the toe stands to strengthen your ankles and calves. This can also restore your stability and balance.

Stand near a sturdy chair or counter. Place your hands on top of the counter and use it for balance. Do not lean too much on the counter.

Push your feet off the floor and stand at the balls of your feet. Count for few seconds then lower your feet. Breathe regularly throughout the exercise. Repeat 10 times for each foot.

Finger marching

This exercise can strengthen your grip and upper body muscles. It can also improve your arm, shoulder and back flexibility.

Stand with your feet firmly on the floor. Imagine a wall in front of you and walk your fingers up the wall until they are above your head. Hold for few seconds then walk back down.

Next, bring both of your hands to your back and reach for both elbows using opposite hands. Hold the position for few seconds. Release your hold and stretch them in front of you. Weave your fingers in front of you and push your hands away from your body. Make sure that your palms are facing away from your body.

Stage 2: Moderate

Move on to the second stage if you have been doing the stage 1 exercises for at least 2 weeks. Add these exercises to those of stage 1.

Biceps curls

Bicep curls can strengthen your arms significantly and help you perform basic arm range of motion.

Hold a light weight in each hand then sit in a chair. Place your feet flat on the floor and your palms should be facing your thighs. Count to two then lift the weights to your shoulders while keeping your upper arm and elbow close to your body. Make sure that your wrists are straight. Repeat the movement 10 times. Do not allow your elbows to move away from the body.

Step ups

This is a great exercise to strengthen your legs, buttocks and hips. It can also help you improve your balance.

You can use the handrail for balance. Make sure to plant your feet firmly on the floor. Walk up the first step, make sure that your knee is straight and it should not move pass your ankle. Use one leg to hold your weight then lower the other foot on the floor. Do not allow your back leg to do all the work.

Overhead press

This exercise can target several muscles in your body at the same time including your upper body, shoulders and arms. It can also strengthen your upper arms.

Stand behind a chair and place your feet shoulder width apart on the floor. Hold a weight on each hand and raise it to shoulder level. Make sure that your palms are facing forward. Pause, then push your arms above your head until they are fully extended. Don't let the weights move too far in front or behind you. Repeat the movement 10 times.

Hip abduction

This exercise targets the muscles in the thighs, buttocks and hips. This can make your hips less vulnerable to fracture.

Stand behind a chair with your feet slightly apart and your toes forward. Keep your legs straight but avoid locking your knees. Count to two then lift your one leg to the side. Make sure that your leg is straight. Pause for a second then lower your leg. Repeat 10 times then repeat on the other side.

Stage 3: Advanced

Make sure that you are comfortable in doing stages 1 and 2 before moving on to the third stage. Add these exercises to the first two sets.

Knee extension

This exercise targets the quadriceps muscles in your thighs. This exercise can strengthen your knees.

Strap on ankle weights and sit in a chair. Make sure that your back is resting all the way back in the chair. Place your feet shoulder width apart. Let your arms rest on your sides. Lift your leg and extend it in front of you. Pause then slowly lower it down to the ground. Repeat 10 times. Rest for a minute then complete the second set.

Knee curl

This is a good exercise to strengthen your upper leg muscles and hamstrings. This can make walking and climbing the stairs easier.

Wear your ankle weights then stand behind a chair. Keep your foot flexed then bend one leg. Bring your heel towards your buttocks. Pause and lower your foot. Do this 10 times and repeat on the other side. Keep your thighs in line at all times.

Pelvic tilt

This exercise can improve your posture and tighten your abdominal muscles. Place a mattress on the floor then lie flat on your back. Bend your knees and place your arms to your side. Roll your pelvis and lift it off the floor. Make sure that your back and shoulders are in place. Pause and lift your pelvis. Repeat 10 times and repeat the movement for a minute.

Floor back extension

The floor back extension is a good exercise if you suffer from weak abdominal muscles. Lie face down on the floor. Place two pillows under your hips and extend your arm straight in front of you. Count to two then lift your arm and leg off the floor. Pause then lower your arm to the floor. Make sure that your head, neck and back is in a straight line. Repeat the exercise 10 times. Perform two sets.

Stage 4: Difficult

These exercises should only be performed if you can do stage 3 exercises with ease.

Abdominal curl

Strengthening your abdominal muscles can improve your stability and helps correct your posture. Lie on your back with your knees bent. Make sure that your feet are flat on the floor. Place your hands behind your head. Raise your shoulders and back off the floor. Pause and lower your body. Repeat 10 times. You can rest for one minute then perform another set.

Chest press

This exercise strengthens the shoulders and chest. Lie on the floor. Bend your knees and hold a light weight in each hand. Lift your arm at shoulder level. The elbows should be slightly bent and make sure that your palms are facing your knees. Straighten your arms above your chest. Lower your arm to your body slowly. Repeat for two sets with 10 repetitions each.

Lunge

Each lunge can strengthen the upper leg and hips. Stand behind a sturdy chair. Hold the chair in front of you for balance. Take a step forward with one leg and bend your knee. Lower your hips towards the floor. Push against the floor and lift your body. Rest for a minute then perform the same exercise on the other leg. Never allow your knees to push past your toes. Keep your body straight.

Upright row

This exercise can strengthen the back muscles and upper arms. Stand with your feet a hip width apart. Hold a weight in each hand with your palms facing your thighs. Bend your elbows and lift your arms in front of you. Raise your elbows slightly higher. Pause before lowering the weights. Repeat 10 times then finish a second set.

Chapter 5. Flexibility and Balance Exercises for People over 60

Stretching and balance exercises can improve your flexibility and give you more freedom of movement. Make sure that you stretch regularly after your cardio and strength training. Make each flexibility exercise last for at least 5 minutes.

Flexibility exercises

Neck stretch

You can choose to stand or sit in a chair. Place your feet on the floor place about shoulder width apart. Turn your head to the right until you feel a light stretching of the muscles. Hold the position for 10 seconds. Turn your head to the left then hold for another 10 seconds.

Shoulder stretch

Stand back against a wall. Your feet should be shoulder width apart. Bend your elbows and make sure that your fingertips are pointing towards the ceiling and your arms touch the wall behind you. Hold for 10 seconds then slowly roll your shoulder forward while keeping your arms bent. Point your palms toward the floor and touch the wall again. Hold for another 10 minutes.

Shoulder and upper arm rise

Stand with your feet apart. Hold one end of a towel with your one hand. Bend your arm to drape the towel on your back. Reach behind you and grasp the other end with your other arm. Stretch your shoulder by pulling the towel down with your one arm. Reverse the movement and repeat 5 times.

Upper body stretch

Stand facing the wall. You should be an arm's length away from the wall. Lean your body forward and place your hand flat against the wall on chest level. Make sure that your back is straight. Slowly walk your hands up the wall until it is above your head. Repeat 5 times.

Chest stretch

Perform this stretch while standing or sitting down. Keep your feet on the floor and place them apart. Stretch your arms to the sides with your palms facing forward. Move your arms back and make sure to squeeze your shoulders together. Hold the position for 30 seconds then return to starting position.

Ankle stretch

Sit in a sturdy chair. Extend your legs in front of you. Tilt your foot and make sure that your heels are on the floor. Bend your ankles towards your body. Hold for 10 seconds then repeat on the other leg.

Back of leg stretch

Lie on the floor with your back straight. Raise one leg but keep the knee slightly bent. Hold your leg with your hands. Make sure that your back is flat against the floor. Hold the position for 10 seconds then repeat with the other leg.

Thigh stretch

Lie on one side. Keep your legs together and lay your head on one arm. Bend the top knee and hold with one hand. Gently pull until you feel a slight strain. Hold the position for 10 seconds. Repeat the movement 5 times. Repeat the exercise on the other leg.

Hip stretch

Lie flat on your back with your knees slightly bent. Keep your legs together and lay your feet on the floor. Your shoulders should also remain on the floor throughout. Lower one of your knees while keeping your feet together. Lower it as far as you can without moving the other knee. Hold the position for 10 seconds then bring it back up. Repeat 3 times with each leg.

Lower back stretch

Lie on your back and keep your knees together. Bend your legs slightly while keeping your feet firmly on the floor. Lower both your legs to one side and hold for few seconds. Bring your legs back up then repeat it on the other side. Alternate the movements on each side.

Calf stretch

Stand in front of a wall then place both of your palms flat against it. Step one foot forward and bend the knee until you feel the stretch at the back of your calf muscles. Hold for few seconds then stand back up. Repeat the exercise with the other leg. Alternate the movement on each leg.

Balance exercises

Standing on one foot

Stand up behind a chair. Hold on to it for balance. Lift one foot while slightly bending your knee. Hold the position for 10 seconds. Do the same thing on the other leg. Repeat 10 times with each leg.

Walking heel to toe

Place one foot in front of the other. One heel should touch the toes of the other foot. Take one step by placing your heel just in front of your other foot's toe. Take about 20 steps. Make sure that you are not looking down while performing this exercise. It is best if you focus on one spot in front of you to keep you steady while you walk.

Balance walking

Raise your arms to the side about shoulder length. Look straight ahead to keep your balance. Walk in a straight line by placing one foot in front of the other. Make sure that you lift your back leg as you walk. Walk slowly and pause for a second before taking another step.

Back leg raises

Hold a chair in front of you to keep your balance. Breathe in slowly as you lift one leg to your back without bending your knees. Do not lean forward. The standing leg should be slightly bent. Hold the position for a second and lower your leg. Repeat the exercise 15 times on each leg.

Side leg rises

Stand behind a chair with your feet slightly apart. Use the chair for balance. Breathe out and lift one leg and extend it to the side. Make sure to keep your back straight and your toes facing forward. Slightly bend the leg you are currently standing on. Hold for a second then lower your leg. Repeat the exercise for 15 times on each leg.

Chapter 6. Yoga for People over 60

Yoga exercises have become very popular in many states. It has inspired entrepreneurs to establish many fitness centers, develop equipment, design clothing and even promote an entire lifestyle. Yoga can be very beneficial for seniors since it can relieve fatigue, stress and pain. Most importantly, yoga is a kind of exercise that can make you feel younger.

Mountain pose

Benefits: Better breathing, improves posture and mental clarity

Stand with your feet apart to ensure that your weight is evenly spread. Place your arms at your sides. Breathe in deeply at an even pace. You can place your hands in a prayer position or extend it overhead to reach up to the sky.

Downward facing dog

Benefits: Improves blood circulation, strengthens heels and calf muscles

Place your feet and hands on the ground while keeping your buttocks pointing to the sky. Slowly walk your hands farther from each other. Make sure to slightly bend your knees. You can get a better stretch if you keep your heels on the ground while alternately pressing your feet down.

Warrior pose

Benefits: Strengthens the leg muscles

Stand with your legs wide apart. Turn your right foot to a 90 degree angle. Extend your arms to the sides while keeping your shoulders down. Lunge your right knee while bending the other leg slightly. Keep your right knee over your foot and don't allow it to go past your toes.

Tree pose

Benefits: Improves your balance, strengthens the spine

Start with the mountain pose then shift your weight in one leg. Keep your hips forward and place one sole on your other leg. Make sure to find your balance. Bring your hands together in a prayer position. Repeat the movement on the other side.

Bridge pose

Benefits: Strengthens the chest, spine and neck. This is a good warm up for more intense back workouts.

Lie on the floor and place your arms at your side. Press the feet into the floor and bend your knees slightly. Slowly lift your hips to the ceiling. Bring both of your hand under your back for support. Lift your hips until they are parallel to the floor. Bring your chin to your chest.

Triangle pose

Benefits: Stretches the body, relieves backache and strengthens the knees

Start with the warrior pose without lunging into your knees. Touch the inside of your right foot with your right hand. Stretch your left hand to the ceiling. Turn your head forward and stare past your left hand.

Seated twist

Benefits: Gives the body a full stretch after a long day sitting.

Sit on the floor and extend your legs in front of you. Cross the right foot over the left leg. Bend the left knee and keep the right knee pointed upward. Place your right hand on the floor for balance. Place the left elbow on the outside of the right knee. Twist to the right side as far as you can.

Upward facing dog

Benefits: Lie face down on the floor. Your thumbs should be just under your shoulders. Extend your legs on the floor. Push your hips down as you squeeze your glutes. Lift your chest off the floor and slightly tilt your head upward. Hold the position for few seconds then relax.

One-legged wind releasing pose

Benefits: Provides a gentle stretch for the middle and lower back and relieves muscle pain.

Lie on the floor and bend your knees. Hold your right thigh close to your chest. Straighten the left leg and remember to keep your foot flexed. Keep your right side and pelvis on the floor. You can also bend your left leg slightly. Hold the position and take few breathes. Repeat on the other side.

Staff pose

Benefits: This position strengthens your back muscles and improves your posture.

Sit on the floor and stretch your legs in front of you. Contract your core and straighten your back. Place your hands in front of you with your fingers pointing towards your toes. Flex your thigh muscles and press it to the floor. Rotate it inward and pull your groin muscles to your tailbone. Flex the ankles and point the toes towards the body. Hold the position for 10 seconds then relax.

Garland pose

Benefits: Great for the hips and can be a good exercise after spending too much time sitting down in a chair.

Stand with your feet apart then bend your knees and come to a squat. You can turn your toes outside if necessary. Place your hands together in prayer position in front of you. Your arms should be placed slightly forward than your knees.

Lunge position

Benefits: This is a great stretch for your legs and back muscles

Straighten your legs and place your feet back under your hips. Extend your left leg back for a deep lunge. Bring your bent leg over your ankle and make sure that your leg is parallel to the floor. Make sure that the extended leg is straight. Hold for five seconds before switching to the other leg.

Plank position

Benefits: Strengthens the arm and back muscles.

Start with the lunge position with your left foot extended at your back. Slowly extend your right leg and place it beside your other leg. This is the basic position before you do a push-up. You can slightly bend your elbows if it becomes too uncomfortable.

Chapter 7. Exercise with Equipment for People over 60

Resistance band exercises

Resistance bands are popularly used for strength training. It is great equipment for people over 60 who wish to work out in their homes. Using resistance bands can help strengthen your muscles and improve your range of motion.

Overhead arm raises

Benefits: Strengthens the shoulders and arms which can increase your mobility.

Step on one end of the resistance band to keep it secure. Hold the other end with your right hand. Bend your elbow slowly towards your back. Keeps your elbow pointing upward with your right hand behind your back. Straighten your arm and extend it towards the sky. Hold the position for few seconds then lower your arm. Repeat it on the other arm.

Knee extensions

Benefits: This exercise can strengthen your hamstrings and upper leg muscles

Sit on a chair then tie one end of the resistance band on one leg for support. Bend the knees at a 90 degree angle. Slowly straighten your knee as far as you can against the resistance band. Slowly bend your knee. Relax and repeat this on the other knee

Neck strengthening exercise

Benefits: This exercise can relive neck pain and fatigue. It also targets upper back muscles.

Wrap the band around the back of your head then hold both ends in front of you. Bend the elbows and slowly extend your arms forward. Make sure to keep your neck straight. Slightly bend your elbows then repeat the movement.

Bicep curls

Place the middle of the band under your feet and hold both ends with your hands. Place your arms to your sides. Gently bend your elbow while keeping the wrists straight. Lift your hands to your shoulders. Slowly relax your arm then repeat on the other arm.

Seated hip flexion exercise

Benefits: Helps ease lower back pain and increases flexibility on the hips

Sit in a chair and wrap the resistance band around your lower thigh. Step on one end of the band with your right leg. Bend your knees slightly then lift your left foot off the ground. Lift your foot as high as you can then hold the position for few seconds. Lower your foot then repeat with the other leg.

Stability ball exercises

Using stability balls can help strengthen your core and improve your balance. It creates an unstable surface and forces you to move in certain ways to maintain your balance.

Pelvic circles

Benefits: Strengthens your lower back and enables you to move your lower body independent from your back.

Sit on the ball and keep your posture neutral. Place your feet firmly on the ground. Slide your hips to the right to move the ball to the right. Do the same thing to your left side. Keep your shoulders steady as much as possible.

Leg drops

This strengthens your hip flexors and leg muscles

Start the exercise by lying on your back. Place your legs on top of the ball and bend your knees to 90 degrees. Roll the ball downward to lower your leg. Slowly return to the starting position. Repeat the same movement on the other leg.

Back extension

Benefits: Strengthens the back and core muscles

Set the ball on the floor then lie face down on it. Rest your hands on the side of the ball. Slowly raise your upper body off the ball while keeping your elbows at 90 degrees. Lower your arms and chest.

Rolling plank

Benefits: Strengthens abdomens, hips and shoulders

Kneel in front of the stability ball then place your forearms on top of it. Tighten your core and straighten your arms to move the ball. Breathe normally as you use controlled movements. Continue to push forward until your elbows are fully extended. Get back to the starting position and repeat the movement.

Ab crunch

Benefits: Strengthens the core muscles

Lie on the stability ball. Make sure that the ball is in the middle of your spine. Place your arms to the side with your fingers pointing to your knees. Keep your knees apart. Lift your shoulders to your knees. Use your core to pull your body up.

Chapter 8. Tips for Exercising

Exercise should be part of your daily routine. This not only makes you healthier but also makes you feel younger as well. Here are some tips in getting the most out of your work out.

Safety tips

Anyone who is new to physical exercise should practice enough caution. Make sure to contact your health care provider before you start any program. You can also ask your doctor about the exercises that you can do. Ask your doctor about any signs like chest pain, irregular heart beat and joint pain which may mean that you need to stop working out as well as the right time to exercise in relation to taking your medications.

Generally, people who are over 60 years of age should not work out too intensely if they find it difficult to talk or breath. However, a little soreness in the muscle is normal and should not prevent you from continuing.

Have a solid plan

You can see better results and stay motivated for a longer time if you make a plan and try to stick to it.

Start where you are

If you have been staying active most of your life, then you would probably know your strengths and weakness when it comes to working out. However, if it has been a while since you last exercised it is important that you start with small activities and gradually increasing the duration and intensity of work outs when you are ready.

Increase your heart rate at your own pace

Getting your heart rate to 50-85% of your maximum heart rate (220 minus your age) is the best way to improve your heart rate and deliver oxygen and blood to your muscles. The idea of high intensity exercise may be daunting for seniors but keep in mind that high intensity is relative to your own fitness level and should not be compared to someone who is 20 years younger than you. Start with three sessions consisting of 15 minutes of high intensity cardio each week.

Do not neglect warm-up, cool-down and stretches

Older people can experience problems with their joints, tendons and ligaments. These problems can worsen if you do not properly prepare your muscles for the exercise. Stretching exercises can also improve your flexibility and increase your range of motion.

Be creative and remember to have fun

Enjoying your workouts is very important. Anything that can keep you moving like dancing, gardening or even walking the dog can be a fun and enjoyable workout.

Tips in working out for free

Joining a commercial fitness center is not the only way to get fit. Here are some tips in working out for free.

Work out at home

Exercising at home is one of the cheapest ways to get fit. You can do basic moves like jumping jacks and crunches at home. You can even do this while watching TV or waiting for the dishes to dry. If you do not own any weights, you can use 1 liter water bottles as an alternative.

Exercise DVDs

Many libraries have a collection of fitness videos which you can barrow. These DVDs can provide helpful instructions in your work out. It's like having your own trainer in your own home. Make it more enjoyable by inviting the family to join in.

Community programs

Most communities and states promote free fitness programs. These can include morning yoga programs at local parks or free swimming lessons. Take advantage of these programs and call your local parks and recreation department to find out the specific schedule.

Playing sports with children

Playing any sport with your grandchildren can also be a cardio exercise. Schedule a weekend to play with them at the park. This can also serve as a great opportunity to bond with your family.

Take advantage of the outdoors

The cheapest exercise is walking. Instead of using the treadmill, try to look for a scenic route near your area to work out in. The fresh air can also be beneficial to your health. Cycling outdoors is also a good and cheap alternative to gym cardio programs.

Tips in building the exercise habit

You should be consistent if you want to build a habit in exercising.

Set a time

Deciding when you are going to work out makes it more likely for you to stick with the schedule. If you have enough time in the morning, you can take a 30 minute stroll around the block before you start your day. If you are not a morning person, you can schedule your exercise at the evening right before you eat dinner.

Use a reminder

If you tend to lose track of your appointments, you can use a form of reminder like a memo note or even a phone reminder so that you will not forget your exercise appointment.

Progress

Give your body enough time to adapt to your new exercise routine. Wait for at least two weeks before increasing the intensity of your work outs. You know that you are ready for a more difficult work out if your old routine seems too easy already.

Make it enjoyable

Do not associate working out with physical discomfort and look at it as an opportunity to have fun instead. This way, you can look forward to doing it. You can enjoy the fresh air in the morning or enjoy the scenery.

Lay out your gear

The fewer obstacles there are, the more likely you are to succeed. Lay out your workout clothes and equipment the night before and place it in near your bed so that when you wake up you will be instantly reminded to work out.

Mix it up

Having a variety of activities to try can make it more exciting. Also, doing a variety of exercises can work different muscles every work out session. Aside from getting a full body work out, you are also giving your muscles enough time to recover.

Train with someone

Having someone to work out with you can give you the necessary motivation to continue your program.

Chapter 9. Frequently Asked Questions

Why do my feet numb when I use pedals?

Many people can experience numbness in their feet while using pedaled machines like the elliptical machine or stationary bicycles. Some people may find this as a minor problem and may be caused by being in constant contact with a pedal. You can minimize the discomfort by wearing cushioned shoes. You can also try pedaling forward and backward every few minutes. Also, try short, high intensity workouts instead of long elliptical workouts.

Is it safe to wear ankle weights while walking?

Fitness experts discourage the use of ankle weights while doing general daily activities. You can still increase your risk of injury even if they are light weights. Wearing weights can alter your normal movements and do not provide the body that much of a benefit anyway. Use your ankle weights to do stationary leg exercises instead.

My hands and feet swell during my workout, is it normal?

The swelling of hands and feet is considered normal in the sense that it is not caused by any medical condition. It will usually disappear after you're done with your exercise. If you continue to experience swelling along with other symptoms like pain and redness, you should already check with your doctor to see if you have medical problems.

Can I exercise if I have asthma?

Exercise is actually beneficial for people with asthma. However, you should contact your doctor to develop a good fitness plan that can work for you to reduce the risk of attack. Work with a medical professional and try to keep the intensity low for the first few days. Once you experience asthma symptoms, reduce your intensity level but you can still continue with the exercise. You can also use your inhaler before your work out session to reduce the risk of asthma attack.

Do ankle wraps and knee braces keep my joints safe during my work out?

Braces and supportive devices can be helpful for people over 60 because they can support your joints. These wraps and braces are also being used when recovering from an injury. Braces can support the joints and give you stability. However, your main goal should be to strengthen your joints so that they can support themselves without any braces. Try to use braces only if they are truly needed otherwise try stretching exercises instead to strengthen your joints.

Is it okay to exercise if I have a cold?

It is very important to listen to your body when deciding if it is okay to exercise. If you are unwell do not push your body pass its limits. It is okay to take a rest from any physical activity until it clears up.

Should I do cardio or strength training first?

It is ideal to do these exercises on different days so that you can devote your time and effort on each one. However, if it is not possible for you to do that then you should think about your goals. If you plan to increase your muscle mass then start with light cardio and focus more on muscle exercise. If your overall fitness goal is to lose weight then focus on cardio exercises more.

What is weight loss plateau and how do I overcome it?

Weight loss plateau occurs when your body stops losing weight even if you are still continuing your fitness program. You will eventually hit a plateau once your body starts to adapt to your fitness routine. You can start increasing the intensity and duration of your exercise and altering your diet to start losing weight again.

What is interval training?

Interval training is alternating between high intensity exercises and periods of active rest. As you progress, you can decrease the amount of rest time and increase the intensity. Seniors are only recommended to perform one interval training per week until they are used to it.

How much exercise should I do?

Most doctors and fitness experts recommend 30 to 60 minutes of exercise each day. However, studies show that you do not even have to work out that long to reap the benefits of physical exercise. Studies show that 30 minutes of activity can reduce your risk of stroke, high blood pressure and heart disease.

Should I lift weights?

Even people over 60 can manage to lift small weights. Lifting weights can help you lose weight and keep it off. It can also strengthen your muscles and enable you to perform daily chores much easier. The stronger your muscles are, the better you will be at performing aerobic exercise. Gaining muscle can also help you look younger and better.

What is BMI and it is useful?

BMI or Body Mass Index is a method of estimating a person's body fat based on their weight and height. It can be helpful in estimating your healthy weight range using BMI. However, one of its limitations includes overestimating the fat percentage of overweight and obese people.

Chapter 10. Glossary of terms

A

Aerobic exercise

It is an activity where your muscles move in a rhythmic manner for a long period of time. Aerobic exercise can drastically improve your cardiovascular fitness. Most common form of aerobic exercise includes running, cycling, swimming and walking.

B

Balance

Balance is a component of physical fitness which involves the maintenance of your body's equilibrium while in movement or in a standard position.

Balance exercise

This is a set of movements that are designed to improve your balance and withstand different physical challenges from destabilizing stimuli and postural imbalance caused by self movement and other external objects.

BMI

BMI or body mass index is the measurement of body fat in relation to height and weight.

C

Calories

A calorie is a unit of energy that is consumed through food and beverages. It is usually burned through various physical activities.

Cardio exercise

Cardio exercise is any activity that can increase your heart rate by at least 50% of its maximum capacity. Cardio exercise can be used interchangeably with aerobic exercise.

Cognitive decline

Cognitive decline is a mental impairment that is described as having trouble remembering things. It can also affect a person's ability to learn new things and make sound decisions.

Coordination

Coordination is the ability to use different parts of the body simultaneously and effectively.

D

Duration

Duration is the total amount of time which the activity is performed. This is usually stated in minutes.

Weight

Weight is strength training equipment with a short bar for handle. Both ends are attached with weights. This is typical equipment used for increasing muscles mass.

E

Energy

This is the strength required to perform physical and mental activities.

Exercise

This is a type of physical activity that is structured and repetitive. It is usually done with a purpose like improvement of physical state or maintenance of a healthy weight.

F

Flexibility

This is a physical fitness component that is described as the ability to perform a range of motion using a specific joint. Flexibility depends on various factors like tightness of the tendons and ligaments.

Frequency

Frequency is the number of times that a certain activity is being performed. This is usually expressed in session or times per week.

H

Health

Health is the condition of being able to perform physical, social and psychological activities. Positive health is usually associated with the capacity to engage in multiple activities with ease while negative health is associated with disease and premature death.

Hormone

Hormone is a substance produced in the body and is transported in the organs through body fluids. Hormones play an important role in keeping the body functioning well.

I

Injury

Injury refers to the damage inflicted on the body. It prevents the body from functioning in normal condition.

Intensity

Intensity is the magnitude of an activity being performed. In layman's term, it is the range of how difficult an exercise is.

Immunity

Immunity is the body's ability to resist infection and toxin.

L

Lifestyle changes

This is a term used to describe the changes that a person implements in their daily routine. A lifestyle change can be positive or negative.

M

Memory

It is describes the brain's ability to store and remember certain information.

Muscle

This is a bundle of tissues that has the ability to produce movements and maintain a certain shape for the body.

Moderate intensity

In the scale of physical activity, moderate intensity refers an activity that is done 3 times of the intensity of rest.

P

Physical activity

This is a range of body movements that requires the contraction of skeletal muscles that increases energy expenditure above normal heart rate.

Physical fitness

Physical fitness describes the body's ability to carry out different activities with vigor and agility.

Progression

Progression is increasing the intensity, frequency and amount of activity in general as the body starts to adapt to a certain pattern.

S

Stamina

Stamina is the body's ability to perform an activity for a long period of time.

Strength

Strength is the ability of the muscles to exert force.

Stretching exercise

Stretching exercise is a form of physical exercise where the muscles are strategically flexed and stretched to improve its elasticity and to achieve a better muscle tone.

W

Weight training

Weight training is a physical activity that involves lifting weights to build muscles.

Conclusion

Thank you again for downloading this book!

I hope this book was able to help you exercise safely.

The next step is to try these exercises for yourself.

Finally, if you enjoyed this book, please take the time to share your thoughts and post a review on Amazon. It'd be greatly appreciated!

Thank you and good luck!

Printed in Great Britain
by Amazon